Commission on information and accountability for
Women's and Children's Health

KEEPING PROMISES, MEASURING RESULTS

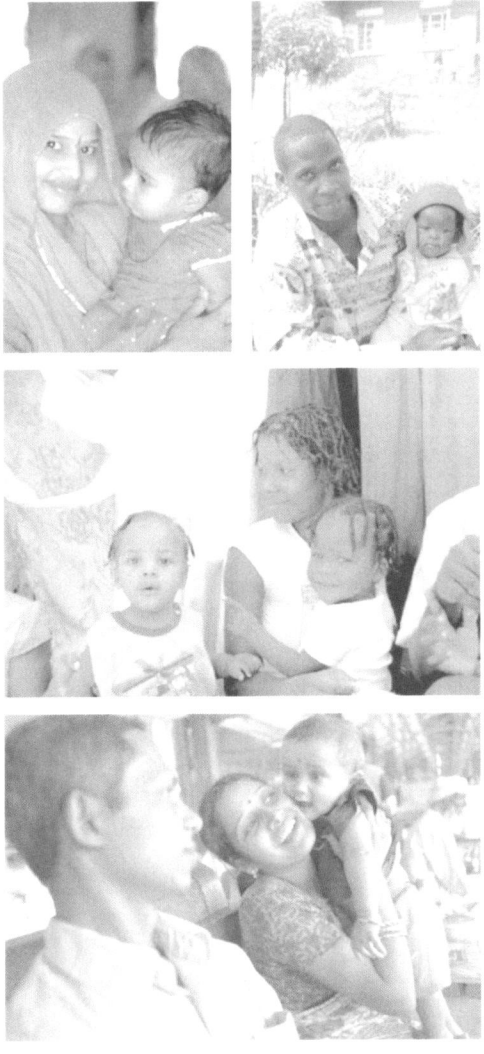

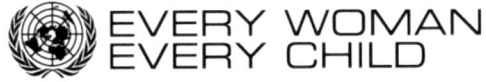

WHO Library Cataloguing-in-Publication Data

Keeping promises, measuring results: Commission on information and accountability for Women's and Children's Health.

1.Women's health. 2.Child welfare. 3.Millennium development goals. 4.Health status disparities. 5.Poverty. 6.Social responsibility. 7.International cooperation. 8.Interinstitutional relations. I.Commission on Information and Accountability for Women's and Children's Health.

ISBN 978 92 4 156432 8 (NLM classification: WA 310)

© World Health Organization 2011

All rights reserved. Publications of the World Health Organization are available on the WHO web site (www.who.int) or can be purchased from WHO Press, World Health Organization, 20 Avenue Appia, 1211 Geneva 27, Switzerland (tel.: +41 22 791 3264; fax: +41 22 791 4857; e-mail: bookorders@who.int). Requests for permission to reproduce or translate WHO publications – whether for sale or for noncommercial distribution – should be addressed to WHO Press through the WHO web site (http://www.who.int/about/licensing/copyright_form/en/index.html).

The designations employed and the presentation of the material in this publication do not imply the expression of any opinion whatsoever on the part of the World Health Organization concerning the legal status of any country, territory, city or area or of its authorities, or concerning the delimitation of its frontiers or boundaries. Dotted lines on maps represent approximate border lines for which there may not yet be full agreement.

The mention of specific companies or of certain manufacturers' products does not imply that they are endorsed or recommended by the World Health Organization in preference to others of a similar nature that are not mentioned. Errors and omissions excepted, the names of proprietary products are distinguished by initial capital letters.

All reasonable precautions have been taken by the World Health Organization to verify the information contained in this publication. However, the published material is being distributed without warranty of any kind, either expressed or implied. The responsibility for the interpretation and use of the material lies with the reader. In no event shall the World Health Organization be liable for damages arising from its use.

This publication contains the report of the Commission on information and accountability for Women's and Children's Health and does not necessarily represent the decisions or policies of the World Health Organization.

HE Ban Ki-Moon
Secretary-General, United Nations
1 United Nations Plaza
New York, NY 10017

May 31, 2011

Excellency,

It is with great pleasure as Co-chairs of the *Commission for Information and Accountability for Women's and Children's Health* that we convey to you the final report of the Commission, on behalf of all Commissioners, Vice-chairs, and other stakeholders engaged in this process.

The *Commission* was convened by the World Health Organization at your request, in order to "determine the most effective international institutional arrangements for global reporting, oversight and accountability on women's and children's health". We believe that the successful adoption and implementation of the recommendations of the *Commission* by all stakeholders will act as a force multiplier for your *Global Strategy for Women's and Children's Health*, and for achieving the Millennium Development Goals by 2015.

Commissioners came together from a broad range of backgrounds, including governments, international organizations, civil society, foundations, academia, and the private sector, to work toward a common cause: to improve the health of women and children. The *Commission* studied the challenges and obstacles that have led to limited progress on improving maternal health, and prevented better progress on reducing child mortality. Lack of capacity for collecting and analysing data, and tracking resources allocated to health, particularly maternal, newborn and child health, weak civil registration systems, and duplication of efforts are some of the issues that have hampered progress.

Commissioners reached consensus on the need to take bold action to accelerate progress. In undertaking this work, they embraced the principles articulated by the *Global Strategy*, particularly:

- focusing on national leadership and ownership of results, as countries themselves are the foundation of accountability;
- strengthening and harmonizing existing country, regional and global-level mechanisms to build on existing efforts and avoid the proliferation of new initiatives; and
- linking accountability for resources to the results, outcomes and impacts they produce.

The *Commission's* ten recommendations focus on improving information for better results, improving tracking of resources, and stronger oversight of both results and resources at national and global levels.

In order to be successful in our commitment to improving the lives of women and children, we are inviting all stakeholders to join us in continuing to work together to improve accountability for resources and results linked to women's and children's health. We encourage them to integrate the principles of the *Global*

Strategy and the *Commission* into their work, and urge them to implement these recommendations, including the prioritization of the 11 core indicators recommended by the *Commission*.

These 11 core indicators on health outcomes and coverage were selected because they align with the indicators for the Millennium Development Goals and with the continuum of care for maternal, newborn, and child health. As well, indicators for resource tracking will allow for better monitoring of the impact those resources have on the lives of women and children.

The *Commission* aimed to clarify and consolidate the current landscape in order to help accelerate progress for women's and children's health in a way that is inclusive, equitable, and sustainable. We can work smarter if we work together.

With regard to institutional arrangements, the *Commission's* report supports building upon and providing incentives to strengthen current institutional mechanisms in order to increase the impact of existing efforts. A small group of independent experts, supported by a small secretariat within the WHO will be charged with reviewing progress in the implementation of the Commission's recommendations. We encourage your office to work quickly, in consultation with the WHO, to start the selection process and to appoint experts for this group, so that they are equipped to take up their work early in 2012.

As we quickly approach the one year anniversary of the launch of your *Global Strategy*, we must work together to build awareness and mobilize support for this initiative. Outreach and engagement on the Commission's recommendations must align with other efforts made on behalf of the *Global Strategy*, in order to reinforce and build on the progress that has already been made.

We hope that the *Commission's* practical and action-oriented recommendations find momentum within the international community and unite us in fulfilling the moral imperative to improve the lives of the world's most vulnerable women and children.

Please accept, Excellency, the assurances of our highest considerations.

H E Jakaya Mrisho Kikwete
President, United Republic of Tanzania

Rt. Hon. Stephen Harper
Prime Minister of Canada

Executive summary

Of the eight Millennium Development Goals (MDGs), the two specifically concerned with improving the health of women and children are the furthest from being achieved by 2015. They are in urgent need of innovative and strategic actions, supported by political will and resources for greater impact. In September 2010, in an effort to accelerate progress, the Secretary-General of the United Nations launched the *Global Strategy for Women's and Children's Health*. The main goal of this strategy is to save 16 million lives by 2015 in the world's 49 poorest countries. It has already mobilized commitments estimated at US$ 40 billion. However, commitments need to be honoured, efforts harmonized, and progress tracked. Actions need to address results and resources.

Given that accountability for financial resources and health outcomes is critical to the objectives of the *Global Strategy*, the Secretary-General asked the Director-General of the World Health Organization to coordinate a process to determine the most effective international institutional arrangements for global reporting, oversight and accountability on women's and children's health.

The work of the Commission on Information and Accountability for Women's and Children's Health is built on the fundamental human right of every woman and child to the highest attainable standard of health and on the critical importance of achieving equity in health. All accountability mechanisms should be effective, transparent and inclusive of all stakeholders. In addition, the Commission's work has embraced the *Global Strategy*'s key accountability principles:

- focus on national leadership and ownership of results;
- strengthen countries' capacity to monitor and evaluate;
- reduce the reporting burden by aligning efforts with the systems countries use to monitor and evaluate their national health strategies;
- strengthen and harmonize existing international mechanisms to track progress on all commitments made.

Accountability begins with national sovereignty and the responsibility of a government to its people and to the global community. However, all partners are accountable for the commitments and promises they make and for the health policies and programmes they design and implement.

The accountability framework's three interconnected processes – monitor, review and act – are aimed at learning and continuous improvement. The framework links accountability for resources to the results, outcomes and impacts they produce. It places accountability soundly where it belongs: at the country level, with the active engagement of governments, communities and civil society; and with strong links between country-level and global mechanisms.

The Commission's 10 recommendations

Ten recommendations have been agreed by all Commissioners. They focus on ambitious, but practical actions that can be taken by all countries and all partners. Wherever possible, the recommendations build on and strengthen existing mechanisms.

Better information for better results

1. **Vital events: By 2015, all countries have taken significant steps to establish a system for registration of births, deaths and causes of death, and have well-functioning health information systems that combine data from facilities, administrative sources and surveys.**

2. **Health indicators: By 2012, the same 11 indicators on reproductive, maternal and child health, disaggregated for gender and other equity considerations, are being used for the purpose of monitoring progress towards the goals of the *Global Strategy*.**

3. **Innovation: By 2015, all countries have integrated the use of Information and Communication Technologies in their national health information systems and health infrastructure.**

Better tracking of resources for women's and children's health

4. **Resource tracking: By 2015, all 74 countries where 98% of maternal and child deaths take place are tracking and reporting, at a minimum, two aggregate resource indicators: (i) total health expenditure by financing source, per capita; and (ii) total reproductive, maternal, newborn and child health expenditure by financing source, per capita.**

5. **Country compacts: By 2012, in order to facilitate resource tracking, "compacts" between country governments and all major development partners are in place that require reporting, based on a format to be agreed in each country, on externally funded expenditures and predictable commitments.**

6. **Reaching women and children: By 2015, all governments have the capacity to regularly review health spending (including spending on reproductive, maternal, newborn and child health) and to relate spending to commitments, human rights, gender and other equity goals and results.**

Better oversight of results and resources: nationally and globally

7. **National oversight:** By 2012, all countries have established national accountability mechanisms that are transparent, that are inclusive of all stakeholders, and that recommend remedial action, as required.

8. **Transparency:** By 2013, all stakeholders are publicly sharing information on commitments, resources provided and results achieved annually, at both national and international levels.

9. **Reporting aid for women's and children's health:** By 2012, development partners request the OECD-DAC to agree on how to improve the Creditor Reporting System so that it can capture, in a timely manner, all reproductive, maternal, newborn and child health spending by development partners. In the interim, development partners and the OECD implement a simple method for reporting such expenditure.

10. **Global oversight:** Starting in 2012 and ending in 2015, an independent "Expert Review Group" is reporting regularly to the United Nations Secretary-General on the results and resources related to the *Global Strategy* and on progress in implementing this Commission's recommendations.

The work of the Commission has concluded with this report. To realize the accountability framework for women's and children's health set out here, all stakeholders must take bold and sustained action as part of their own work as well as collectively through collaboration on the *Global Strategy*. We urge all stakeholders to remain ambitious, and to channel their aspirations into implementing our recommendations.

We believe the framework, the recommendations and the actions we have set out are the best ways to ensure that the commitments pledged though the *Global Strategy* make a tangible difference in the lives of women and children. While the scope of the Commission relates to women's and children's health, the framework is relevant to health more broadly and, thus, could serve as a catalyst for strengthened accountability within national health systems and across the global health community.

" All partners are accountable for the promises they make and the health policies and programmes they design and implement. Tracking resources and results of public health spending are critical for transparency, credibility and ensuring that much-needed funds are used for their intended purposes and to reach those who need them most. Ultimately, the recommendations made by this Commission are about improving the health – and indeed saving the lives of women and children around the world. "

Jakaya Kikwete, President of the United Republic of Tanzania

1. Introduction

The world is making important progress in reducing the number of women and children dying from preventable causes. In the past two decades there has been a steady decline in child deaths, from an estimated 11.9 million in 1990 to 7.7 million in 2010; and, according to recent estimates, the number of women dying in childbirth fell by one third from over half a million in 1990 to about 350,000 by 2008. Although many low-income countries remain off-track to meet the Millennium Development Goals for maternal and child health, it is not too late for the goals to be attained.

> "The Commission has developed bold yet practical measures that will help save the lives of mothers and children living in the world's poorest countries. Through our collective efforts we will ensure tangible progress in achieving our goals, but only if we remain fully committed to making the recommendations in this report a reality."
>
> Stephen Harper, Prime Minister, Canada

The good news is that progress looks set to accelerate. In 2010, for the first time, the Group of Eight (G8) and the African Union summits focused on maternal and child health. The African Union launched a coordinated campaign to be delivered by the African Union Commission. In September 2010, the United Nations General Assembly discussed the theme in a special event at which the Secretary-General launched the *Global Strategy for Women's and Children's Health* (*Global Strategy*). The main objective of this strategy is to save 16 million lives by 2015 in the world's 49 poorest countries. It has already mobilized commitments estimated at US$ 40 billion from governments, philanthropic institutions, the United Nations and multilateral organizations, civil society and nongovernmental organizations, the business community, health-care workers and professionals, and academic and research institutions around the world.

In spite of these positive developments, success will be achieved only if all stakeholders take concerted actions. Commitments need to be honoured, efforts integrated and progress tracked more actively. Actions need to address results and resources. The absence of civil registration systems in low- and middle-income countries, and the resulting weakness of vital statistics on births, deaths and causes of death, has hampered efforts to build a reliable evidence base from which health improvement can be measured. In addition, the management of health systems is often weak and impedes direct measurement of achievements towards the health-related MDGs. There is also a lack of adequate universal instruments for accurately tracking both national and international financial commitments to women's and children's health and subsequent disbursements in countries.

All stakeholders agree on the importance of having a new, robust accountability framework to ensure that available resources and results are identified, recognized, reviewed and reported on in order to more rapidly improve women's and children's health.

Accountability is essential. It contributes to ensuring that all partners honour their commitments, demonstrates how actions and investment translate into tangible results and better long-term outcomes, and tells us what works and what needs to be improved. The Secretary-General, therefore, asked the Director-General of the World Health Organization (WHO) to coordinate a process to determine the most effective international institutional arrangements for global reporting, oversight and accountability on women's and children's health.

The time-limited Commission on Information and Accountability for Women's and Children's Health (the Commission) comprises leaders and experts from Member States, multilateral agencies, academia, civil society and the private sector. Our deliberations and recommendations have been informed by two expert working groups, one on accountability for results, the other on accountability for resources. We have also taken into consideration a background paper on information and communication technologies (ICTs), country case-studies and public comments on the draft reports of the two working groups submitted through the Commission's web site and online discussion forum. This report and all the inputs that went into its development, including the two working group reports, are available at (www.everywomaneverychild.org/accountability_commission).

> *"Timely, reliable and accessible health information is critical for accountability. Having this solid information at country level is essential to measuring and monitoring results. One of our top priorities must be investing in helping countries build the capacity needed to capture this health information – that means giving them the financial and technical resources required to monitor things such as births, deaths and causes of deaths and achieve the accountability revolution needed to save women and children from dying."*
>
> Dr Margaret Chan, Director-General of the World Health Organization

Although the *Global Strategy* focuses on the 49 lowest-income countries, our framework aims to apply to all countries and stakeholders. Where relevant, we focus certain recommendations on the 74 countries that account for more than 98% of maternal and child deaths. Furthermore, while we recognize the significance of other health determinants and sectors, such as education, water and sanitation, in improving the health of women and children, our recommendations focus specifically on the health sector. We focus on the immediate policy objective – accelerating progress towards the MDGs for women and children, notably MDGs 1c, 4 and 5.[a] We welcome the positive impact that innovation is having on improving health outcomes. Innovation is needed broadly in science and technology development (e.g. medicines, vaccines and medical devices), social and behavioural change, and in the delivery of interventions, including business models that stimulate private sector investment in women's and children's health. However, our report concentrates specifically on the innovative use of ICTs to provide more accurate and timely data for monitoring and reviewing results and resources for women's and children's health.

In this, our final report, we fulfil all of our objectives. We have proposed a framework that places accountability soundly where it belongs: at the country level, with the active engagement of national governments, parliaments, communities and civil society. We also make strong links between country-level and global mechanisms and holding donors accountable. Ten recommendations have been agreed by all Commissioners. They focus on ambitious, but practical actions that can be taken by all countries and all development partners, including civil society, private foundations and the corporate sector.

[a] 1c. Halve, between 1990 and 2015, the proportion of people who suffer from hunger; 4. Reduce by two thirds, between 1990 and 2015, the under-five mortality rate; 5a. Reduce by three quarters the maternal mortality ratio; 5b. Achieve universal access to reproductive health.

2. The accountability framework

The foundations of the accountability framework (Fig. 1) are built on the fundamental human right of every woman and child to the highest attainable standard of health and on the critical importance of achieving equity in health and gender equality. Women's and children's health is recognized as a fundamental human right in such treaties as the International Covenant on Economic, Social and Cultural Rights; the Convention on the Elimination of All Forms of Discrimination against Women; and the Convention on the Rights of the Child. The Human Rights Council also recently adopted a specific resolution on maternal mortality. The goal of the framework is to ensure that the most off-track Millennium Development Goals, for maternal and child health, are met by 2015.

Fig. 1. **The accountability framework for women's and children's health**

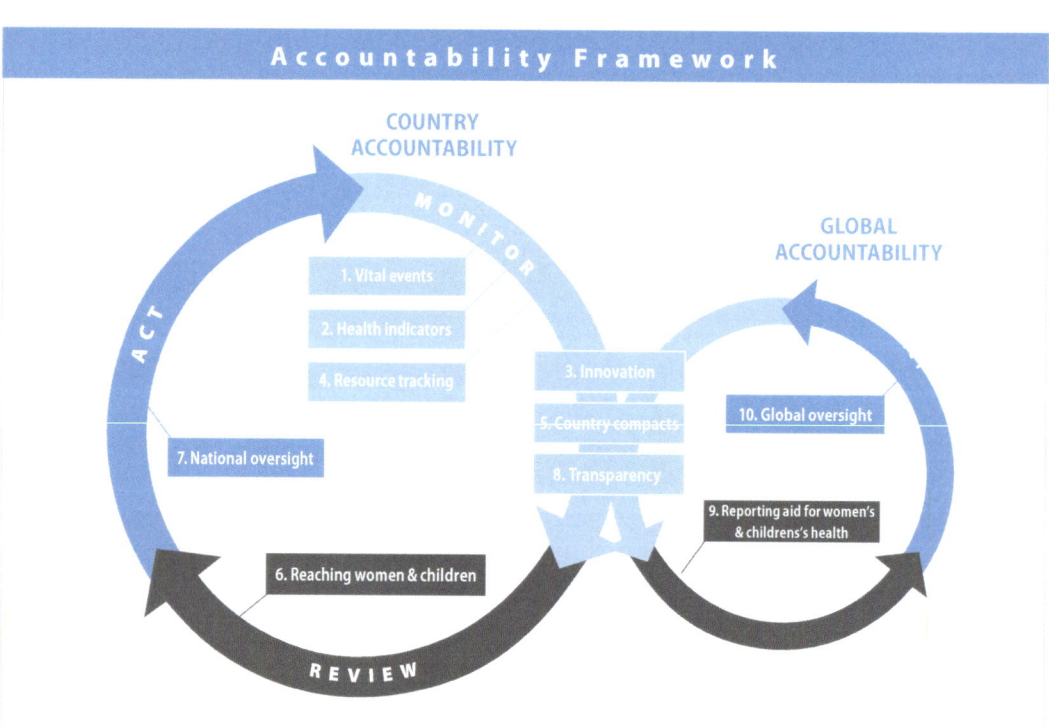

The urgent need for collective action is clear.

In addition, the framework embraces the *Global Strategy*'s key accountability principles:

- focus on national leadership and ownership of results;
- strengthen countries' capacity to monitor and evaluate;
- reduce the reporting burden by aligning efforts with the systems countries use to monitor and evaluate their national health strategies;
- strengthen and harmonize existing international mechanisms to track progress on all commitments made.

Accountability begins with national sovereignty and the responsibility of a government to its people and to the global community. However, all partners are accountable for the promises they make and the health policies and programmes they design and implement.

National accountability mechanisms are more likely to be effective if they are selected by countries, rather than directed from outside, and fit their specific circumstances. The accountability framework assumes that mechanisms will be nationally or locally selected, with strong legitimacy and high-level political leadership, and be effective, transparent and inclusive of policy, technical, academic, professional and civil society constituencies.

The accountability framework covers national and global levels and comprises three interconnected processes – monitor, review and act – aimed at learning and continuous improvement. It links accountability for resources to results, i.e. the outputs, outcomes and impacts they produce.

Monitor means providing critical and valid information on what is happening, where and to whom (results) and how much is spent, where, on what and on whom (resources).

Review means analysing data to determine whether reproductive, maternal, newborn and child health has improved, and whether pledges, promises and commitments have been kept by countries, donors and non-state actors. This is a learning process that involves recognizing success, drawing attention to good practice, identifying shortcomings and, as required, recommending remedial actions.

Act means using the information and evidence that emerge from the review process and doing what has been identified as necessary to accelerate progress towards improving health outcomes, meeting commitments, and reallocating resources for maximum health benefit. This includes more support for and wider adoption of policies and programmes that are having a positive impact, and taking action to address what is not working, remedying problems with data, weak practices and any mismatch between actual resources and promises. It also includes learning from best practices and experience to enhance the effectiveness of efforts to improve women's and children's health.

Most countries already have some sort of monitor-review-act system in place, and these should be built on and strengthened. In most countries, the focus must be on strengthening and aligning such accountability mechanisms. In several countries these systems are extensive and include subnational review processes as an integral part of national reviews, broad stakeholder participation and consultation, and involvement beyond the health sector. Box 1 below highlights elements of the monitor-review-act accountability framework in Ghana, Rwanda and the United Republic of Tanzania.

While the immediate scope of the Commission relates to women's and children's health, the framework is relevant to health more broadly and, thus, could serve as a catalyst for strengthened accountability within national health systems and across the whole global health community.

Box 1. The accountability framework in countries

Ghana, Rwanda and the United Republic of Tanzania have developed their own systems of monitoring, review and action, based on many years of experience with sector-wide approaches in health. In general, these approaches help to ensure that the health-sector strategy is linked with broader development goals and planning processes, notably national strategies for economic growth and poverty reduction. There is also a consistent link between reviews and resource allocation through medium-term expenditure frameworks and annual operational planning cycles, and there are subnational processes of review and action.

National **monitoring** of progress and performance as part of health-sector strategic plans focuses on a core set of indicators: 18 in Rwanda, 37 in Ghana and 40 in the United Republic of Tanzania. Reproductive, maternal, newborn and child-health indicators account for at least half of these core indicators; they are also core indicators in the monitoring component of overall development plans.

Data availability and quality have improved during the past decade, mostly because of more frequent health surveys. The monitoring inputs in annual reviews, however, are mostly based on facility and administrative sources, which are affected by persistent problems with the timely availability and quality of data. The completeness, timeliness and quality of the data are areas all three countries are looking to improve with the aid of Information and Communication Technologies (ICTs). In Rwanda, the facility and administrative reporting systems appear to be improving significantly as a result of developing an overall architecture, introducing ICTs, and using performance-based funding. Reliable and timely data on births and deaths and causes of death are lacking in all three countries. In general, more systematic investments are needed to improve the performance of the national health information system, ensuring that a reliable and transparent monitoring system is in place.

The **institutional mechanisms** to support critical elements of monitoring (including data generation, compilation and sharing, quality assessment, analysis and synthesis, and communication of results) need considerable strengthening in all three countries. These functions tend to be concentrated in the Ministry of Health, with limited capacity in staff manpower and skills. Involving key country institutions and independent assessment should be integral parts of the monitoring process. In Ghana, independent consultants from within and outside the country are contracted to prepare the annual review report. In the United Republic of Tanzania, the review is mostly prepared by the Ministry of Health and Social Welfare, with inputs from national institutions. In Rwanda, although no formal report synthesizes all monitoring data for the reviews, performance-based funding and the use of ICTs are leading to greater transparency and data access.

Health-sector **reviews** and planning summits are conducted on at least an annual basis, with broad stakeholder involvement. Reproductive, maternal, newborn and child-health reviews are embedded in the well-established processes. Development partner participation is prominent, but civil society's role is less clear. Monitoring and evaluation subcommittees of the health sector committee involve multiple stakeholders. Many but not all development partners have aligned themselves with these country-led monitoring and review platforms, which are also promoted as part of the International Health Partnership principles.

In the context of the *Global Strategy,* the three countries have made specific commitments that are a subset of existing country plans for reproductive, maternal, newborn and child health. The *Global Strategy* is perceived as an opportunity to strengthen the implementation of national strategies to accelerate progress towards MDG 4 and particularly MDG 5.

Note: see http://www.everywomaneverychild.org/pages?pageid=14&subpage=69 for the report of the three country case studies.

3. Holding all stakeholders accountable: 10 recommendations

The Commission is making 10 specific, measurable, attainable and time-bound recommendations for implementing the accountability framework, and which highlight the urgent actions needed to overcome the impediments to greater accountability. The recommendations seek better information for better results; better tracking of resources for women's and children's health; and stronger oversight of results and resources, nationally and globally. Progressive target dates acknowledge that countries' capacities vary and that they will move forward at different rates. How the recommendations can be achieved is detailed in the Agenda for Action that follows.

Better information for better results

1. **Vital events: By 2015, all countries have taken significant steps to establish a system for registration of births, deaths and causes of death, and have well-functioning health information systems that combine data from facilities, administrative sources and surveys.**

There can be no accountability without timely, reliable and accessible health information and data. Solid information at the country level is essential to measure and monitor results. A strong capacity in countries to collect data on the health of women and children is essential to determine where investments should be focused and whether progress is being made. Many countries do not have well-functioning, integrated health information systems that combine information from population-based sources, such as surveys, with facility and administrative data. Major efforts are required to move towards one sound country system that meets all data needs for women's and children's health; ICTs provide new opportunities to do so.

The inability to count births and deaths and identify causes of death has been called a "scandal of invisibility" (see Fig. 2). Vital statistics from various sources provide information that benefits individuals, societies and decision-makers. Solutions to these data gaps exist, but building civil registration systems to deliver accurate and reliable data demands long-term political commitment and investment. That kind of political will has been mostly lacking, resulting in the information base for improving women's and children's health being heavily dependent on surveys conducted several years apart. In many countries, these surveys have had significant inputs from outside agencies, such as the Demographic and Health Surveys, and Multiple Indicator Cluster Surveys.

Countries most off-track for women's and children's health generally have the weakest civil registration systems. There is no single blueprint for collecting reliable vital statistics. Each country's challenges are unique, so solutions must be tailored to circumstances and needs. Investments must be channelled into data-gathering, together with the human and institutional capacities to support such systems.

> *"With mobile connectivity now widespread in even the world's poorest countries, ICTs offer a unique and powerful opportunity to bridge the health development gap. In addition to facilitating data gathering, sharing and analysis, platforms like the Internet and social media can also be used as tools to create safe and empowering spaces for women, where they can obtain accurate, up-to-the-minute health information in a confidential, multilingual environment."*
>
> Dr Hamadoun Touré, Secretary-General, International Telecomunication Union

Fig. 2. **Health information situation in the 49 lowest-income countries[a] listed in the *Global Strategy***

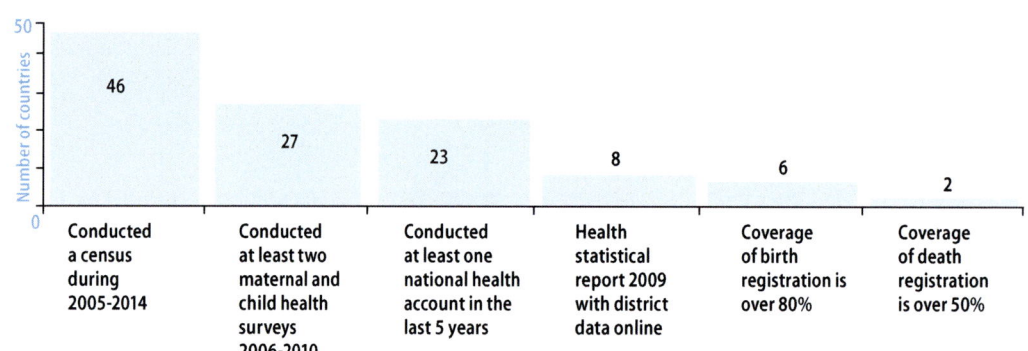

Adapted from: *Country health information systems: a review of the current situation and trends.* Geneva: World Health Organization and Health Metrics Network; 2011.
[a] United Nations least developed countries (http://unstats.un.org/unsd/methods/m49/m49regin.htm#least, as of 17 February 2011).

ICTs have great potential to help countries overcome persistent obstacles in developing birth and death registration systems and rapid reporting of vital events. Liberia, for example, is experimenting with using mobile phones to register births. Together with WHO and other partners, the Health Metrics Network is looking to revitalize the monitoring of vital events through innovative information technology solutions (MOVE-IT for the MDGs), combined with a periodic report describing the state of the world's information systems for health.

2. **Health indicators: By 2012, the same 11 indicators on reproductive, maternal and child health (see Box 2), disaggregated for gender and other equity considerations, are being used for the purpose of monitoring progress towards the goals of the *Global Strategy*.**

The 11 indicators of women's and children's health should be reported for the lowest wealth quintile, gender, age, urban/rural residence, geographic location and ethnicity; and, where feasible and appropriate, for education, marital status, number of children and HIV status.

In addition, the Commission urges countries to monitor the quality of care that women and children – boys and girls alike – receive, especially in the poorest countries. Quality means safe and effective care that is a positive experience for the user. Subnational data should also be collected as they are especially important for a complete assessment of equity and the right to health of all women and children.

Box 2. The 11 indicators of maternal, newborn and child health

One set of indicators has been selected to monitor the status of women's and children's health:

- maternal mortality ratio (deaths per 100 000 live births);
- underfive child mortality, with the proportion of newborn deaths (deaths per 1000 live births);
- children under five who are stunted (percentage of children under five years of age whose height-for-age is below minus two standard deviations from the median of the WHO Child Growth Standards).

These three health status indicators are essential for monitoring MDGs. Stunting, a nutrition indicator, is important for understanding not only outcomes, but also determinants of maternal and child health. Nutrition is also a useful proxy indicator for development more broadly.

These indicators are relatively insensitive to change and do not show progress over short periods (in the absence of birth and death registration systems they can only be measured with substantive time lags). Therefore, more sensitive and timely data that can monitor almost real-time changes in a set of key interventions to improve women's and children's health are needed. This objective can be achieved by monitoring a tracer set of eight coverage indicators:

- met need for contraception; (proportion of women aged 15-49 years who are married or in union and who have met their need for family planning, i.e. who do not want any more children or want to wait at least two years before having a baby, and are using contraception);
- antenatal care coverage (percentage of women aged 15–49 with a live birth who received antenatal care by a skilled health provider at least four times during pregnancy);
- antiretroviral prophylaxis among HIV-positive pregnant women to prevent vertical transmission of HIV, and antiretroviral therapy for women who are treatment-eligible;
- skilled attendant* at birth (percentage of live births attended by skilled health personnel);
- postnatal care for mothers and babies (percentage of mothers and babies who received postnatal care visit within two days of childbirth);
- exclusive breastfeeding for six months (percentage of infants aged 0–5 months who are exclusively breastfed);
- three doses of the combined diphtheria, pertussis and tetanus vaccine (percentage of infants aged 12–23 months who received three doses of diphtheria/pertussis/tetanus vaccine);
- antibiotic treatment for pneumonia (percentage of children aged 0–59 months with suspected pneumonia receiving antibiotics).

These eight coverage indicators have been selected because they are strategic and significant: each one represents a part of the continuum of care and each one is connected with other dimensions of health and health systems. A measure of contraception is needed as a tracer for reproductive health. Antenatal care provides a measure of access to the health system and is critical to ensuring proper coverage of care to identify maternal risks and improve health outcomes for the mother and newborn. HIV-related indicators are included to emphasize the need to move towards a more holistic approach to health care, and to encourage further integration of health services. Skilled birth attendance, postnatal care and breastfeeding are critical elements of the continuum of care. The recommended vaccine is delivered routinely and so helpfully measures a child's ongoing interaction with the health system. Finally, case management of childhood pneumonia is an indicator of access to treatment. Although a vaccine will have a long-term impact on pneumonia, case management will remain an important measure of success.

These 11 indicators have been selected from a combination of the 11 MDG indicators and the 39 indicators used by the Countdown to 2015 for Maternal, Newborn and Child Survival. The Commission endorses the use of both sets of indicators. However, although all countries monitor and report on a large number of health indicators, updates on health status indicators are often based on predictions and there are major gaps in the availability of recent data to assess progress. Therefore, the Commission has recommended a small subset of 11 core indicators to ensure the collection of consistent and timely data needed to hold governments and development partners accountable for progress in improving women's and children's health, without adding to countries' reporting requirements. Reducing the reporting burden – i.e. duplicative reporting requirements – is a priority for the Commission and low-income countries. Collecting better information will be easier if scarce resources in countries are allocated to do so; this approach includes having all partners focus their efforts and reporting requirements around these indicators.

*A skilled attendant is an accredited health professional — such as a midwife, doctor or nurse — who has been educated and trained to proficiency in the skills needed to manage normal (uncomplicated) pregnancies, childbirth and the immediate postnatal period, and in the identification, management and referral of complications in women and newborns. *Making pregnancy safer: the critical role of the skilled attendant: A joint statement by WHO, ICM and FIGO.* World Health Organization, 2004. http://whqlibdoc.who.int/publications/2004/9241591692.pdf

3. Innovation: By 2015, all countries have integrated the use of Information and Communication Technologies in their national health information systems and health infrastructure.

ICTs can help enormously to disseminate and share information on results and resources for women's and children's health. ICTs provide new possibilities to capture and process data, link information systems, increase the timeliness of information produced, and store data for institutional memory. Constructing patient records, collecting data remotely, and transmitting those data for central storage and analysis are a few examples of the practical benefits of ICT systems, which allow for clear and rapidly accessible audit trails of administrative and financial transactions. Combining Internet and mobile communications also supports data collection directly from individuals and health facilities in remote and rural areas, and enables that data to be shared in a timely and equitable manner (see Box 3). Improved storage and access at public databases will enhance transparency. New methods and information will be more easily shared, and participation in the review process expanded. Social networking offers fresh opportunities for strengthening accountability mechanisms, while broadband technologies can accelerate connectivity between community, national and global levels, and progress towards generating, synthesizing and sharing comprehensive health information for improving women's and children's health.

Box 3. Using mobile phones to collect health data

Many pilot projects around the world have experimented with using mobile phones to collect health data. In Senegal, for example, the Ministry of Health improved data collection by equipping community health workers in 10 districts with hand-held devices and data collection software. The benefits included more frequent supervision visits in the pilot areas, faster data collection and analysis (one district reported that data that took two weeks to collect on paper was collected in one hour), and the use of data by health officials to reallocate budgets.

Source: Mobilizing maternal health: Senegal's use of EpiSurveyor for maternal health data collection based on an evaluation by Dalberg Development Advisors.

The use of e-health and m-health should be strategic, integrated and support national health goals. In order to capitalize on the potential of ICTs, it will be critical to agree on standards and to ensure interoperability of systems. Health information systems must comply with these standards at all levels, including systems used to capture patient data at the point of care. Common terminologies and minimum data sets should be agreed on so that information can be collected consistently, easily shared and not misinterpreted. In addition, national policies on health-data sharing should ensure that data protection, privacy and consent are managed consistently.

The potential applications for ICTs are as diverse as ICTs themselves, and must be employed at every opportunity for a more complete understanding of patient care, including patients' own understanding of the services to which they are entitled.

Better tracking of resources for women's and children's health

4. **Resource tracking: By 2015, all 74 countries where 98% of maternal and child deaths take place are tracking and reporting, at a minimum, two aggregate resource indicators: (i) total health expenditure by financing source, per capita; and (ii) total reproductive, maternal, newborn and child health expenditure by financing source, per capita.**

Tracking resources is critical for transparency, credibility and ensuring much-needed funds are used for their intended purposes and reach those who need them most. Parliaments have an important role to play in holding governments accountable for such reporting The long-term objective is for governments to annually report on their total health expenditure from all financing sources, (including the government, private entities such as firms and individual households and development partners) and for specific health priorities, such as maternal health, malaria and HIV, or population groups (women and children, for example). To this end, countries, starting with those with the greatest burden of women's and children's mortality and morbidity, should receive development partner support to strengthen their capacity to track and report on these two aggregate resource indicators.

Fig. 3. **Country capacity for producing national health accounts, (NHA) 2011**

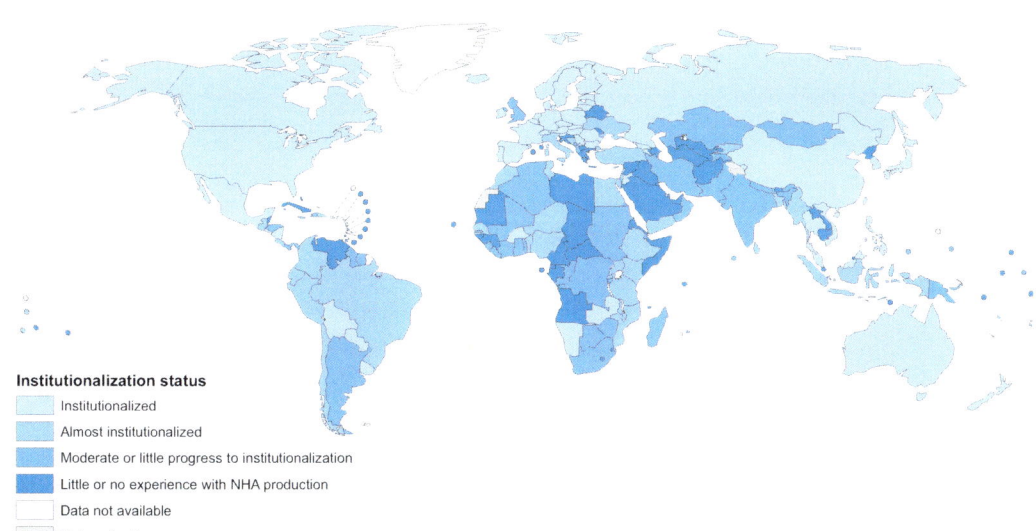

Monitoring expenditures on health, and more specifically on women's and children's health, is not done on a systematic basis. Many low-income countries do not have the capacity to routinely produce expenditure estimates (Fig. 3). The Commission recognizes that countries are starting with different capacities to track resources and will need to progressively expand their reporting of health expenditures over time. If necessary, countries can start by annually tracking total government health expenditure and external assistance, and providing more detailed reporting on private sources as their capacity increases. All stakeholders will have a role to play in providing timely and accurate information to governments to enable a comprehensive understanding of available resources and their use.

Tracking expenditure on women's and children's health stretches the capacities of many countries. Rapid and simple estimation methods need to be further developed by WHO and the Organisation for Economic Co-operation and Development for use by countries with limited capacity.

To enable countries to achieve this target, their capacity to track resources for health, organize data into established accounting frameworks, and analyse and use information in national policy and accountability processes needs to be strengthened. Capacity is lowest in low-income countries. Efforts to build this capacity should be made as part of longer-term efforts to strengthen underlying public expenditure management systems.

5. **Country compacts: By 2012, in order to facilitate resource tracking, "compacts" between country governments and all major development partners are in place that require reporting, based on a format to be agreed in each country, on externally funded expenditures and predictable commitments.**

In most countries, agreements, or compacts, between governments and all major development partners can be integrated into existing mechanisms, such as joint financing arrangements, International Health Partnership compacts, memoranda of understanding, and codes of conduct. They are necessary to ensure all partners provide governments with their budget and expenditure reports in an agreed format, thereby reinforcing mutual accountability and giving a clear picture of external health financing and the linkages with national health priorities. Monitoring such agreements via scorecards will further help to ensure compliance.

As part of these agreements, all major development partners (including bilateral donors, private foundations, corporations and nongovernmental organizations) operating within a country should be required to report annually and in a coordinated manner on both the volume and purpose (including reproductive, maternal, newborn and child health) of their health expenditures. They should also provide predictable forward plans, based on a format to be agreed in each country, to the relevant government ministry. Regional and international organizations provide forums that can empower countries to take this step and encourage all development partners to participate.

Development partners should also report their development assistance for health against the aid effectiveness indicators developed through the Paris Declaration and Accra Agenda for Action in order to demonstrate that their funding and programmes for women's and children's health are aligned with country priorities, strategies and planning cycles. Resource flows should also be reviewed to understand the quality of the assistance provided, including how much reaches the country and can be programmed at the country level.

6. **Reaching women and children: By 2015, all governments have the capacity to regularly review health spending (including spending on reproductive, maternal, newborn and child health) and to relate spending to commitments, human rights, gender and other equity goals and results.**

This recommendation is for reviewing resource flows in countries. Initially, countries with less capacity might be able to review only annual government health expenditures. As capacity increases, all countries should make annual reviews of health spending from all financing sources.

First, countries should review spending against priorities budgeted in national (and, where appropriate, subnational) health plans. Ideally, this entails an annual analysis of total health expenditure and its distribution across priority diseases, such as HIV, and population groups (e.g. women and children). Countries should also review country-level data on external resources that have been received for comparison with similar information provided by development partners to the Creditor Reporting System managed by the Organisation for Economic Co-operation and Development. Connecting global-level information to national-level information is critical to understanding the amount and nature of external resources available for use at country level. To this end, all major providers of external resources should sign into the country compacts and consider reporting their assistance to the Creditor Reporting System.

Second, countries should review whether investments are equitably distributed and directed to communities of concern to improve the health of women and children. This entails disaggregating indicators by sex, socioeconomic status and other demographic or geographic variables to reveal inequities in the financial burden and use of services among population groups. Such analyses can inform assessments of whether governments are meeting their commitments to ensuring the right to health.

Third, countries should compare overall public spending on health with results achieved and prioritize intervention investments according to effectiveness and the efficient use of available resources. This prioritization should be linked to the level of impact. Impact can be shown through modelling and measured directly. If direct measurements of impact are not feasible, proxy measures can be used. Proxy measures for results, such as three doses of the combined diphtheria, pertussis and tetanus vaccine coverage, or assisted deliveries, can be used to make a general comparison of results achieved with money spent.

In many countries, parliaments have a mandate to perform these review functions. Efforts to strengthen the capacity of countries to direct resources to women and children should involve parliaments.

Better oversight of results and resources: nationally and globally

7. National oversight: By 2012, all countries have established national accountability mechanisms that are transparent, that are inclusive of all stakeholders, and that recommend remedial action, as required.

The time frame of this recommendation is particularly ambitious because national arrangements are the anchor of our international institutional arrangements. Although the nature of these review mechanisms will vary from country to country, they should be transparent and inclusive, ensuring all key stakeholders, including civil society and communities, are well represented. They should consider independent reviews of data. It is also important that national reviews span subnational, district and local levels.

Many countries already regularly review progress and performance in the health sector against country health plans and international goals. The involvement of higher political levels, such as a president's or a prime minister's office, generates better progress on reproductive, maternal, newborn and child health, and helps strengthen crucial political will.

One of several potential options to strengthen review mechanisms in countries is to establish a national commission for women's and children's health. Chaired by a head of state or government, accountable (and reporting) to parliament, inclusive of all relevant government departments, and engaging nongovernmental actors, such a body would operate in a similar manner to national AIDS commissions (see Box 4). Some countries engage a health ombudsperson to increase the independence of the review.

Box 4. Learning from national AIDS commissions

In 2001, the United Nations General Assembly Special Session (UNGASS) on AIDS mobilized countries in an unprecedented way to address the epidemic. Part of the UNGASS response was to create national AIDS commissions as multisectoral coordinating entities to lead and monitor the response. They have facilitated country mobilization around one national strategy, one national authority and one national monitoring system. They engage civil society and have embedded high-level political commitment into the AIDS response.

Although national AIDS commissions are not perfect and do not have formal legal authority, they "have been able to catalyse and spearhead strong leadership and advocacy in support of the national AIDS policy and action frameworks, and to provide effective multisectoral coordination, especially among non-governmental actors and development partners". There may be exceptional opportunities for countries to build on and leverage the success of UNGASS on behalf of women and children.

Source: Morah E, Ihalainen M. National AIDS Commissions in Africa: performance and emerging challenges. *Development Policy Review* 2009, 27:185–214.

One essential function of a national review is to assess whether health gains and investments are equitably distributed. This entails disaggregating all data on the core indicators. The two sets of indicators to monitor resources flows should be disaggregated by sex, socioeconomic status and other demographic or geographic variables to reveal health inequities, and inequities in the financial burden and use of services among population groups. Countries should also periodically review and analyse barriers in access to health services for women, especially young women.

The highest levels of political authority, including national parliaments, should act to ensure the results of the review inform subsequent national plans, together with commitments on budgets, timelines and further accountability measures. It is especially important to invest in strengthening community-level accountability mechanisms. One example is scorecards used by communities to monitor health services.

8. **Transparency: By 2013, all stakeholders are publicly sharing information on commitments, resources provided and results achieved annually, at both national and international levels.**

Information flows between the producers and users of data (e.g. citizens, programme implementers, development partners, academics, researchers, civil society and the media) are insufficient. Databases should be made more user-friendly to encourage wider use of the information.

Accountability requires that information on results and resources is readily accessible to anyone. Parliaments, which oversee the performance of governments, have a particularly important role in ensuring transparency and inclusiveness, and encouraging continued scrutiny, challenge and debate.

Information should flow freely in accordance with information-sharing principles established by the government. Governments and development partners, including private foundations and the corporate sector, should make information on health outcomes and resources spent on health available on a public domain web site. (see Box 5) Transparency in information can drive community, national, regional and global efforts to increase accountability and to assess relative country progress.

Box 5. Using ICTs to track development assistance

Development Loop is an Information and Communication Technology innovation that can track foreign aid to enhance transparency. It enables users to share their project information with others, both online and offline. They can view their projects alongside those of other organizations, or examine indicators, such as poverty rates or maternal mortality. The prototype includes development projects from the World Bank and Asian Development Bank, and allows for citizen feedback. The application uses these layers to create feedback loops that enable the social monitoring of development projects and promote mutual accountability.

Source: http://www.impactalliance.org/ev_en.php?ID=51450_201&ID2=DO_TOPIC

In this context, exercises such as the report being compiled by The Partnership on Maternal, Newborn and Child Health to track commitments made in response to the *Global Strategy* should provide useful and easily accessible baseline data on the financial, policy and programme commitments announced in September 2010. Going forward, all donors should identify the sources and the intermediaries of financial flows when reporting on commitments in order to avoid double-counting.

The greater availability of information will not only raise awareness of women's and children's health, but allow closer scrutiny of whether health improvements are equitable and whether funds are being used responsibly and equitably. Transparency will foster learning and continuous improvement, and more informed decision-making by all partners.

Such transparency can enhance accountability and overall health-system performance, but the capacity to act on such information must be strengthened. Users inside and outside government should be empowered with information on health determinants, equity issues and budgetary constraints, and through guidance on advocacy techniques to enhance their ability to seek changes in budgets or policies.

9. **Reporting aid for women's and children's health: By 2012, development partners request the OECD-DAC to agree on how to improve the Creditor Reporting System so that it can capture, in a timely manner, all reproductive, maternal, newborn and child health spending by development partners. In the interim, development partners and OECD implement a simple method for reporting such expenditure.**

All major development partners, including emerging donors, private foundations and corporate donors, should provide to the global aid database (the Creditor Reporting System of the Organisation for Economic Co-operation and Development) more timely, complete and consistent information on resources for health. Development partners reporting on financial resources devoted to women's and children's health can be a vital complement to countries reporting on their own health expenditures, and help ensure mutual accountability.

Expenditure by development partners on reproductive, maternal, newborn and child health cannot easily be identified from the Creditor Reporting System data, because these services overlap the current system of coding. The Development Assistance Committee of the Organisation for Economic Co-operation and Development should urgently identify ways to improve the reporting system so that expenditure on reproductive, maternal, newborn and child health can be better captured and in a timely fashion. In the interim, development-partner expenditure on reproductive, maternal, newborn and child health can be estimated using methods developed by the G8 in consultation with the OECD.

10. Global oversight: Starting in 2012 and ending in 2015, an independent "Expert Review Group" is reporting regularly to the United Nations Secretary-General on the results and resources related to the Global Strategy and on progress in implementing this Commission's recommendations.

One of the Commission's objectives is to recommend international institutional arrangements for global reporting, oversight and accountability on women's and children's health. Several national and international interagency groups, technical organizations and academic institutions already perform extensive field work and publish regular reports that address many elements of global oversight. They monitor and review different aspects of women's and children's health and recommend action. This work should continue and be strengthened.

The purpose of global oversight is to assess progress in implementing the *Global Strategy* and the recommendations of the Commission in order to accelerate improvements in women's and children's health. The specific functions are to:

- track and ensure all stakeholders honour their commitments to the *Global Strategy* and the Commission; including the US$ 40 billion of commitments made in September 2010, and to track implementation of the recommendations of the Commission;
- assess progress towards greater transparency in the flow of resources and achieving results;
- identify obstacles to implementing both the *Global Strategy* and the Commission's recommendations;
- identify good practice, including in policy and service delivery, accountability arrangements and value-for-money approaches;
- make recommendations to improve the effectiveness of the accountability framework.

However, to provide a stronger accountability mechanism – and to ensure critical remedies and actions are taken – we propose an independent Expert Review Group be established and operate until 2015. This time-limited group would draw extensively on existing data, reporting and assessments at country and global levels, in particular through national accountability frameworks, to avoid duplication, fragmentation and increasing transaction costs through a light process with high impact. The group would synthesize all available information and evidence, address discrepancies, and make its own analysis and recommendations in an annual report to the United Nations Secretary-General.

The key principles underpinning our proposed international institutional arrangements are: partnership, independence, transparency, credibility and efficiency. Networks and partnerships, such as The Partnership on Maternal, Newborn and Child Health, should be used to their maximum potential to promote participation in the review process and in outreach about the Commission's report. The public should also have the opportunity to participate in the review process.

The group should comprise 5-9 members, appointed by the United Nations Secretary-General, with at least half from low- and middle-income countries. There will be broad international representation and diversity of knowledge and experience in the field of women's and children's health. WHO will lead a transparent process to solicit nominations from all of the stakeholders supporting the *Global Strategy*. Nominated individuals will be expected to exercise autonomous, professional judgement and serve in an independent capacity.

The members of the Expert Review Group should be announced in September 2011, the first anniversary of the *Global Strategy*'s launch. A small, well resourced secretariat hosted by WHO should be established to collect data, help prepare reports and provide general support to the group.

4. The Agenda for Action

The work of the Commission has concluded with this report. To realize the accountability framework for women's and children's health set out here, all stakeholders must take bold and sustained action as part of their own work as well as collectively through collaboration on the *Global Strategy*. Recognizing that these actions will build on several existing mechanisms and differing degrees of capacity, we urge all stakeholders to remain ambitious, and to channel their aspirations into the progressive realization of our recommendations. In line with the Commission principles, we propose the following actions be taken at the national and global levels.

At the national level, we urge countries and development partners, to:

- develop roadmaps to strengthen civil registration and the collection of vital statistics supported by innovative ICTs;
- align their results and resources monitoring with the proposed indicators and publicly share the data produced;

- establish or scale up national-level accountability mechanisms, including those of all relevant stakeholders, for national-level review and action on women's and children's health, and to engage civil society and parliamentarians in these efforts;
- strengthen investments in capacity building towards well-functioning health information systems and ensure these investments are made at the national, subnational and community levels.

The H4+ agencies (UNAIDS, UNICEF, UNFPA, WHO and the World Bank) have a special role to play in supporting countries with the least capacity to implement the recommendations.

At the global level, we urge all stakeholders to:

- support countries in their efforts to build capacity to implement our recommendations;
- focus their reporting requirements on the core set of indicators to reduce duplicative reporting requests and to enable countries to better measure progress against Millennium Development Goals 1c, 4 and 5 by 2015 through strengthened health information systems;
- agree on country "compacts", where these do not yet exist, as an important step to reinforce a relationship of mutual cooperation and trust in achieving our shared objectives;
- support efforts by the Organisation for Economic Co-operation and Development to improve the Creditor Reporting System to better capture aid and other external finance aimed at improving reproductive, maternal, newborn and child-health;
- make information on resources pledged and provided, including information on the predictability of commitments, transparent to countries and to the global community, to allow countries to understand total resources available and better manage for results;
- clarify urgently their commitments to the *Global Strategy* and report on progress towards these commitments;
- share information publicly and proactively, including with the Expert Review Group;
- continue to enhance the effectiveness of aid and development assistance for health, including through the monitoring and promotion of the implementation of the Paris Declaration and Accra Agenda for Action commitments in this sector;
- align strategies and mobilize resources to implement the Commission's recommendations;
- provide resources for the functioning of the Expert Review Group, including for the Secretariat.

In addition to national- and global-level actions, the success of the accountability framework depends on strong support from all actors. Uniting actors from all levels of engagement (community, subnational, national, regional and international) around the Commission's accountability framework will build on the unprecedented momentum spurred by the *Global Strategy* and help ensure the Commission's recommendations make a difference in the lives of women and children. In that context, we, the Commissioners:

- commit to continue mobilizing support by personally taking the Commission's recommendations to major national and international forums in order to promote the adoption of recommendations among our peers and stakeholder constituencies;
- look forward to the next meeting of *Global Strategy* partners when implementing the accountability framework will be further discussed. We invite all stakeholders to participate in this event.

5. Conclusion

We believe the framework, the recommendations and the actions set out in this report offer the best means to ensure the commitments pledged though the *Global Strategy* make a tangible difference in the lives of women and children.

We have taken a phased approach to accountability, beginning with a small number of strategic indicators. The assertive monitoring and review of these indicators at national and global levels would catalyse new commitment and action. The history of the HIV response suggests that such a focused approach will deliver broader benefits.

Our framework at country and global levels embeds the monitor-review-act process in national and international arrangements that mirror, support and reinforce one another. We see this country-global alignment with accountability for resources and results – with a common language around the same indicators – as a potentially powerful way to deliver the *Global Strategy*.

The Agenda for Action spells out the steps that need to be taken to better measure results, track resources and report progress, actions recognized by national governments and the global health community as urgent priorities.

We urge the United Nations Secretary-General, national governments, civil society and development partners to act on these recommendations. Doing so will not only benefit women's and children's health, but offer opportunities to integrate wider health priorities within a single accountability framework.

Acknowledgements

The Commission would like to thank the many groups and individuals who contributed to this report, including:

– the two working groups and their chairs; papers are available onhttp://www.everywomaneverychild.org/pages?pageid=14&subpage=20

– the International Telecommunication Union/WHO technical team and their collaborators who contributed a background paper on Information and Communication Technology's contribution to accountability for women's and children's health;

– the WHO case-study teams and the countries that collaborated with them to contribute national-level examples of accountability mechanisms.

Commissioners

Jakaya Mrisho Kikwete (Co-Chair)
President
United Republic of Tanzania
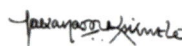

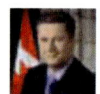
Stephen Harper (Co-Chair)
Prime Minister
Canada

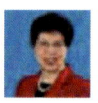
Margaret Chan (Vice-Chair)
Director-General
World Health Organization
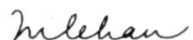

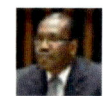
Hamadoun Touré (Vice-Chair)
Secretary-General
International Telecommunication Union
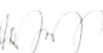

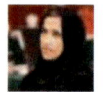
Hessa Sultan Al Jaber
Secretary-General
Supreme Council of Information and Communication Technology, Qatar
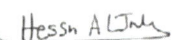

Modou Diagne Fada
Minister of Health
Ministry of Health,
Senegal
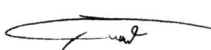

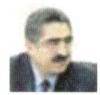
Walid Ammar
Director-General
Ministry of Public Health, Lebanon

Julio Frenk
Chair
Partnership for Maternal, Newborn and Child Health (PMNCH)

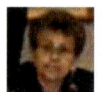
Tamar Manuelyan Atinc
Vice President, Health, Nutrition, and Population
World Bank
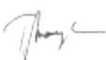

Bience Gawanas
Commissioner of Social Affairs
African Union
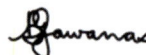

Ghulam Nabi Azad
Minister of Health and Family Welfare
Ministry of Health and Family Welfare, India

Tedros Adhanom Ghebreyesus
Minister of Health
Ministry of Health,
Ethiopia
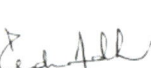

Henri de Raincourt
Minister of Cooperation
Ministry of Foreign and European Affairs, France
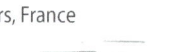

Nyaradzayi Gumbonzvanda
General Secretary
World YWCA
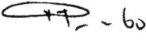

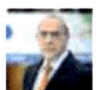
Angel Gurría
Secretary-General
Organisation for Economic Co-operation and Development (OECD)

Peter Piot
Director
London School of Hygiene & Tropical Medicine

Haruna Iddrisu
Minister of Communications
Ministry of Communications,
Ghana

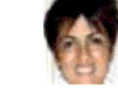
Silvina Ramos
Senior Researcher, Health, Economy & Society Department
Centre of the State and Society (CEDES)

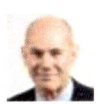
Kevin Jenkins
CEO
World Vision International

Richard Sezibera
Minister of Health
Ministry of Health,
Rwanda

Klaus M. Leisinger
President and Managing Director
Novartis Foundation for Sustainable Development

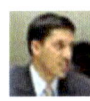
Rajiv Shah
Administrator
United States Agency for International Development (USAID)

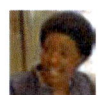
Asha Rose Migiro
Deputy Secretary-General
United Nations (UN)

Jill Sheffield
President
Women Deliver

Andrew Mitchell
Secretary of State for International Development
United Kingdom of Great Britain and Northern Ireland

Jonas Støre
Minister of Foreign Affairs
Department for Humanitarian Affairs,
Norway

Jayaseelan Naidoo
Chairperson
Global Alliance for Improved Nutrition

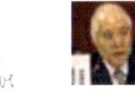
Keizo Takemi
Senior Fellow
Japan Center for International Exchange,
Tokai University

R.M. Marty M. Natalegawa
Minister of Foreign Affairs
Ministry of Foreign Affairs,
Indonesia

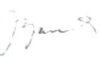
Tachi Yamada
President, Global Health Program
Bill & Melinda Gates Foundation

Annex: Terms of reference

The following are the terms of reference and working procedures for Commissioners serving on the *Commission on Information and Accountability for Women's and Children's Health*:

Background on Commission

Leaders from a wide range of stakeholders including governments, international organizations, civil society, the private sector, foundations and academia have been invited to serve on the *Commission on Information and Accountability for Women's and Children's Health* as Commissioners by Director-General of the World Health Organization (WHO), with the strong support of the United Nations Secretary-General.

Objectives

The *Commission on Information and Accountability for Women's and Children's Health* will propose a framework for global reporting, oversight and accountability on women's and children's health which has the following objectives:

- Determine international institutional arrangements for global reporting, oversight and accountability on women's and children's health. This accountability framework will encompass results and resources, and identify the roles of the different partners involved;
- Identify ways to improve monitoring of progress towards women and children's health, while minimizing the reporting burden on countries, including a core set of indicators, efficient investment in data generation and better data sharing;
- Propose actions to overcome major challenges to accountability at the country level, including strengthening of country capacity and addressing major data gaps, such as the monitoring of vital events;
- Identify opportunities for innovation provided by information technology that will facilitate improved accountability for results and resources, and propose ways of ensuring these opportunities are harnessed to bring maximum benefit to countries.

Scope of Work of the Commissioners

The Commissioners will provide broad policy guidance for the development of the strategic framework for action. The Commissioners will be supported by two Working Groups composed of technical experts. One group will address how to improve accountability for results; the other will address the best way to ensure accountability for financial resources

Timeframe and Modalities

Commissioners shall serve according to their expertise until the delivery of the final report and show a clear commitment to support the Commission. The Commission shall convene at the end of January 2011 and again in late April or early May 2011 in order to complete its final report prior to the meeting of the World Health Assembly in late May 2011.